SWINE FLU

WHAT YOU NEED TO KNOW

The outbreak of disease that be caused by a new influenza virus of swine origin continues to grow in the United States and internationally. Today, the Centers for Disease Control and Prevention (CDC) reports additional confirmed human infections, hospitalizations, and the nation's first fatality from this outbreak. The more recent illnesses and the reported death suggest that a pattern of more severe illness associated with this virus may be emerging in the U.S. Most people will not have immunity to this new virus and, as it continues to spread, more cases, more hospitalizations, and more deaths are expected in the coming days and weeks.

CDC has implemented its emergency response. The agency's goals are to reduce transmission and illness severity, and provide information to help health care providers, public health officials, and the public address the challenges posed by the new virus. CDC regularly issues new interim guidance for clinicians on how to care for children and pregnant women who may be infected with this virus. Young children and pregnant women are two groups of people who are at high risk of serious complications from seasonal influenza. In addition, CDC's Division of the Strategic National Stockpile (SNS) continues to send antiviral drugs, personal protective equipment, and respiratory protection devices to all 50 states and U.S. territories to help them respond to the outbreak.

SWINE FLU

WHAT YOU NEED TO KNOW

EDITED BY

A. M. DUMAR

BROWNSTONE BOOKS

SWINE FLU : WHAT YOU NEED TO KNOW

CONTENTS

WHAT IS A PANDEMIC?

FLU PANDEMICS AND SWINE FLU: A BRIEF HISTORY

ABOUT THE INFLUENZA VIRUS.

PANDEMIC PREPAREDNESS

SWINE FLU: SIGNS, SYMPTOMS, AND DIAGNOSIS

Prevention

Treatment of Swine Flu

Special Instructions for Children

World Health Organization Report on Swine Flu Outbreak

WHAT IS A PANDEMIC?

1. Definition of "Pandemic."

The word "pandemic" comes from the Greek παν (*pan*) meaning "all" and δημοσ (*demos*) meaning "people." It is an epidemic of infectious disease that spreads through populations across a large region, for instance a continent, or even worldwide.

According to the World Health Organization (WHO), a pandemic can start when three conditions have been met:

- Emergence of a disease new to a population.
- Agents infect humans, causing serious illness.
- Agents spread easily and sustainably among humans.

A disease or condition is not a pandemic merely because it is widespread or kills many people; it must also be infectious. For instance, cancer is responsible for many deaths but is not considered a pandemic, because the disease is not infectious or contagious.

2. Pandemics and Notable Epidemics Through History.

There have been a number of significant pandemics recorded in human history, generally zoonoses which came about with domestication of animals, such as influenza and tuberculosis. There have been a number of particularly significant epidemics that deserve mention above the "mere" destruction of cities:

- Plague of Athens, 430 BC. Typhoid fever killed a quarter of the Athenian troops and a quarter of the population over four years. This disease fatally weakened the dominance of Athens, but the sheer virulence of the disease prevented its wider spread — it killed off its hosts at a rate faster than they could spread it. The exact cause of the plague was unknown for many years. In January 2006, researchers from the University of Athens analyzed teeth recovered from a mass grave underneath the city and confirmed the presence of bacteria responsible for typhoid.

- Antonine Plague, 165-180. Possibly smallpox brought to the Italian peninsula by soldiers returning from the Near East; it killed a quarter of those infected, and up to five million in all. At the height of a second outbreak, the Plague of Cyprian (251-266), which may have been the same disease, 5,000 people a day were said to be dying in Rome.

- Plague of Justinian, from 541 to 750, was the first recorded outbreak of the bubonic plague. It started in Egypt, and reached Constantinople the following spring, killing (according to the Byzantine chronicler Procopius) 10,000 a day at its height, and perhaps 40% of the city's inhabitants. The plague went on to eliminate a quarter to a half of the human population that it struck throughout the known world. It caused Europe's population to drop by around 50% between 550 and 700.

- Black Death, started 1300s. Eight hundred years after the last outbreak, the bubonic plague returned to Europe. Starting in Asia, the disease reached Mediterranean and western Europe in 1348 (possibly from Italian merchants fleeing fighting in the Crimea), and killed 20 to 30 million Europeans in six years; a third of the total population, and up to a half in the worst-affected urban areas.It was the first of a cycle of European plague epidemics that continued until the 18th century. During this period, more than 100 plague epidemics swept across Europe. The Third Pandemic started in China in the middle of the 19th century, spreading plague to all inhabited continents and killing 10 million people in India alone.

3. Cholera.

- First cholera pandemic 1816-1826. Previously restricted to the Indian subcontinent, the pandemic began in Bengal, then spread across India by 1820. 10,000 British troops and countless Indians died during this pandemic. It extended as far as China, Indonesia (where more than 100,000 people succumbed on the island of Java alone) and the Caspian Sea before receding. Deaths in India between 1817 and 1860 are estimated to have exceeded 15 million persons. Another 23 million died between 1865 and 1917. Russian deaths during a similar time period exceeded 2 million.

- Second cholera pandemic 1829-1851. Reached Russia , Hungary (about 100,000 deaths) and Germany in 1831, London in 1832 (more than 55,000 persons died in the United Kingdom), France, Canada (Ontario), and United States (New York) in the same year, and the Pacific coast of North America by 1834. A two-year outbreak began in England and Wales in 1848 and claimed 52,000 lives. It is believed that over 150,000 Americans died of cholera between 1832 and 1849.

- Third pandemic 1852-1860. Mainly affected Russia, with over a million deaths. In 1852, cholera spread east to Indonesia and later invaded China and Japan in 1854. The Philippines were infected in 1858 and Korea in 1859. In 1859, an outbreak in Bengal once again led to the transmission of the disease to Iran, Iraq, Arabia and Russia.

- Fourth pandemic 1863-1875. Spread mostly in Europe and Africa. At least 30,000 of the 90,000 Mecca pilgrims fell victim to the disease. Cholera claimed 90,000 lives in Russia in 1866.

- In 1866, there was an outbreak in North America. It killed some 50,000 Americans.

- Fifth pandemic 1881-1896. The 1883-1887 epidemic cost 250,000 lives in Europe and at least 50,000 in Americas. Cholera claimed 267,890 lives in Russia (1892); 120,000 in Spain; 90,000 in Japan and 60,000 in Persia.

- In 1892, cholera contaminated the water supply of Hamburg, Germany, and caused 8606 deaths.

- Sixth pandemic 1899-1923. Had little effect in Europe because of advances in public health, but Russia was badly affected again (more than 500,000 people dying of cholera during the first quarter of the 20th century). The sixth pandemic killed more than 800,000 in India. The 1902-1904 cholera epidemic claimed over 200,000 lives in The Philippines.

- Seventh pandemic 1962-66. Began in Indonesia, called El Tor after the strain, and reached Bangladesh in 1963, India in 1964, and the USSR in 1966.

4. Influenza.

The Greek physician Hippocrates, the "Father of Medicine," first described influenza in 412 BC.

The first influenza pandemic was recorded in 1580, and since then influenza pandemics occurred every 10 to 30 years.

5. Typhus.

Typhus is sometimes called "camp fever" because of its pattern of flaring up in times of strife. (It is also known as "gaol fever" and "ship fever" for its habits of spreading wildly in cramped quarters, such as jails and ships.) Emerging during the Crusades, it had its first impact in Europe in 1489, in Spain. During fighting between the Christian Spaniards and the Muslims in Granada, the Spanish lost 3,000 to war casualties, and 20,000 to typhus. In 1528, the French lost 18,000 troops in Italy, and lost supremacy in Italy to the Spanish. In 1542, 30,000 people died of typhus while fighting the Ottomans in the Balkans.

In the Thirty Years' War, an estimated 8 million Germans were wiped out by bubonic plague and typhus fever. The disease also played a major role in the destruction of Napoleon's Grande Armée in Russia in 1812. Felix Markham thinks that 450,000 soldiers crossed the Neman on 25 June 1812, of whom less than 40,000 recrossed in anything like a recognizable military formation. In early 1813, Napoleon raised a new army of 500,000 to replace his Russian losses. In the campaign of that year, over 219,000 of Napoleon's soldiers were to die of typhus. Typhus played a major factor in the Irish Potato Famine. During the World War I, typhus epidemics killed over 150,000 in Serbia. There were about 25 million infections and 3 million deaths from epidemic typhus in Russia from 1918 to 1922. Typhus also killed numerous prisoners in the Nazi concentration camps and Soviet prisoner of war camps during World War II. More than 3.5 million Soviet POWs died in the Nazi custody out of 5.7 million.

6. HIV and AIDS.

HIV went directly from Africa to Haiti, then spread to

the United States and much of the rest of the world begin-
ning around 1969. HIV, the virus that causes AIDS, is currently a pandemic, with infection rates as high as 25% in
southern and eastern Africa. In 2006, the HIV prevalence
rate among pregnant women in South Africa was 29.1%.
Effective education about safer sexual practices and
bloodborne infection precautions training have helped to
slow down infection rates in several African countries spon-
soring national education programs. Infection rates are rising
again in Asia and the Americas. AIDS could kill 31 million
people in India and 18 million in China by 2025, according
to projections by U.N. population researchers. AIDS death
toll in Africa may reach 90-100 million by 2025.

7. Smallpox.

Smallpox is a highly contagious disease caused by the
Variola virus. The disease killed an estimated 400,000 Europeans each year during the 18th century. During the 20th
century, it is estimated that smallpox was responsible for
300-500 million deaths. As recently as the early 1950s, an
estimated 50 million cases of smallpox occurred in the world
each year. After successful vaccination campaigns
throughout the 19th and 20th centuries, the WHO certified
the eradication of smallpox in December 1979. To this day,
smallpox is the only human infectious disease to have been
completely eradicated.

8. Measles.

Historically, measles was very prevalent throughout the
world, as it is highly contagious. According to the National
Immunization Program, 90% of people were infected with
measles by age 15. Until the vaccine was developed in 1963,
measles was considered to be deadlier than smallpox. In

roughly the last 150 years, measles has been estimated to have killed about 200 million people worldwide. In 2000 alone, measles killed some 777,000 worldwide. There were some 40 million cases of measles globally that year.

Measles is an endemic disease, meaning that it has been continually present in a community, and many people develop resistance. In populations that have not been exposed to measles, exposure to a new disease can be devastating. In 1529, a measles outbreak in Cuba killed two-thirds of the natives who had previously survived smallpox. The disease had already ravaged Mexico, Central America, and the Inca civilization.

9. Syphilis.

Researchers concluded that syphilis was carried from the New World to Europe after Columbus' voyages. The findings suggested Europeans could have carried the nonvenereal tropical bacteria home, where the organisms may have mutated into a more deadly form in the different conditions of Europe. The disease was more frequently fatal than it is today. Syphilis was a major killer in Europe during the Renaissance.

10. Tuberculosis.

One-third of the world's current population has been infected with Mycobacterium tuberculosis, and new infections occur at a rate of one per second. About one in ten of these latent infections will eventually progress to active disease, which, if left untreated, kills more than half of its victims. Annually, 8 million people become ill with tuberculosis, and 2 million people die from the disease worldwide. In the 19th century, tuberculosis killed an estimated one-quarter of the adult population of Europe; and by

1918 one in six deaths in France were still caused by tuberculosis. In the 20th century, tuberculosis killed approximately 100 million people.

11. Leprosy.

Leprosy, also known as Hansen's Disease, is caused by a bacillus, Mycobacterium leprae. It is a chronic disease with an incubation period of up to five years. Since 1985, 15 million people worldwide have been cured of leprosy. In 2002, 763,917 new cases were detected. It is estimated that there are between one and two million people permanently disabled because of leprosy.

Historically, leprosy has affected mankind since at least 600 BC, and was well-recognized in the civilizations of ancient China, Egypt and India. During the High Middle Ages, Western Europe witnessed an unprecedented outbreak of leprosy. Numerous leprosaria, or leper hospitals, sprang up in the Middle Ages; Matthew Paris estimated that in the early 13th century there were 19,000 across Europe.

12 Malaria.

Malaria is widespread in tropical and subtropical regions, including parts of the Americas, Asia, and Africa. Each year, there are approximately 350-500 million cases of malaria. Drug resistance poses a growing problem in the treatment of malaria in the 21st century, since resistance is now common against all classes of antimalarial drugs, with the exception of the artemisinins.

Malaria was once common in most of Europe and North America, where it is now for all purposes non-existent. Plasmodium falciparum became a real threat to colonists and indigenous people alike when it was introduced into the Americas along with the slave trade. Malaria devastated the

Jamestown colony and regularly ravaged the South and Midwest. During the American Civil War, there were over 1.2 million cases of malaria among soldiers of both sides.

13. Yellow Fever.

Yellow fever has been a source of several devastating epidemics. Cities as far north as New York, Philadelphia, and Boston were hit with epidemics. In 1793, the largest yellow fever epidemic in U.S. history killed as many as 5,000 people in Philadelphia—roughly 10% of the population. About half of the residents had fled the city, including President George Washington. Aproximately 300,000 people are believed to have died from yellow fever in Spain during the 19th century. In colonial times, West Africa became known as "the white man's grave" because of malaria and yellow fever.

14. Viral Hemorrhagic Fevers.

Some viral hemorrhagic fever causing agents like Lassa fever, Rift Valley fever, Marburg virus, Ebola virus and Bolivian hemorrhagic fever are highly contagious and deadly diseases, with the theoretical potential to become pandemics. Their ability to spread efficiently enough to cause a pandemic is limited, however, as transmission of these viruses requires close contact with the infected carrier, and the carrier only has a short time before death or serious illness. Furthermore, the short time between a carrier becoming infectious and the onset of symptoms allows medical professionals to quickly quarantine carriers, and prevent them from carrying the pathogen elsewhere. Genetic mutations could occur, which could elevate their potential for causing widespread harm; thus close observation by contagious disease specialists is merited.

15. "Superbugs."

Antibiotic-resistant microorganisms, sometimes referred to as "superbugs," may contribute to the re-emergence of diseases which are currently well-controlled. For example, cases of tuberculosis that are resistant to traditionally effective treatments remain a cause of great concern to health professionals. Every year, nearly half a million new cases of multidrug-resistant tuberculosis (MDR-TB) are estimated to occur worldwide. The World Health Organization (WHO) reports that approximately 50 million people worldwide are infected with multiple-drug resistant tuberculosis (MDR TB), with 79 percent of those cases resistant to three or more antibiotics. In 2005, 124 cases of MDR TB were reported in the United States. Extensively drug-resistant tuberculosis (XDR TB) was identified in Africa in 2006, and subsequently discovered to exist in 49 countries, including the United States. About 40,000 new cases of XDR-TB emerge every year, the World Health Organization estimates.

The plague bacterium could develop drug-resistance and become a major health threat. Plague epidemics have occurred throughout human history, causing over 200 million deaths worldwide. The ability to resist many of the antibiotics used against plague has been found so far in only a single case of the disease in Madagascar.

In the past 20 years, common bacteria including Staphylococcus aureus, Serratia marcescens and Enterococcus, have developed resistance to various antibiotics such as vancomycin, as well as whole classes of antibiotics, such as the aminoglycosides and cephalosporins. Antibiotic-resistant organisms have become an important cause of healthcare-associated (nosocomial) infections (HAI). In addition, infections caused by community-acquired strains of methicillin-resistant Staphylococcus aureus (MRSA) in otherwise healthy individuals have become more frequent in recent years.

16. SARS.

In 2003, there were concerns that Severe Acute Respiratory Syndrome (SARS), a new and highly contagious form of atypical pneumonia, might become pandemic. It is caused by a coronavirus dubbed SARS-CoV. Rapid action by national and international health authorities such as the World Health Organization helped to slow transmission and eventually broke the chain of transmission. That ended the localized epidemics before they could become a pandemic. However, the disease has not been eradicated. It could re-emerge. This warrants monitoring and reporting of suspicious cases of atypical pneumonia.

FLU PANDEMICS AND SWINE FLU: A BRIEF HISTORY.

1. WHAT IS SWINE FLU?

Swine influenza (also called swine flu) refers to influenza caused by any strain of the influenza virus endemic in pigs (swine). Strains endemic in swine are called swine influenza virus (SIV).

Of the three genera of human flu, two also appear in swine: *Influenzavirus A* is common and *Influenzavirus C* is rare. *Influenzavirus B* has not been reported in swine. Within Influenzavirus A and Influenzavirus C, the strains affecting swine and humans are largely distinct.

Swine flu is common in swine and rare in humans. People who work with swine, especially people with frequent close-up exposures, are at risk of catching swine influenza if the swine carry a strain able to infect humans. However, these strains infrequently circulate between humans as SIV rarely mutates into a form able to pass easily from human to human. In humans, the symptoms of swine flu are similar to those of influenza and of influenza-like illness in general: chills, fever, sore throat, muscle pains, severe headache, coughing, weakness, and general discomfort.

The 2009 flu outbreak in humans is due to a new strain of Influenza A virus subtype H1N1 (a notation that refers to the configuration of the hemagglutinin and neuraminidase proteins in the virus) that derives in part from human influenza, avian influenza, and two separate strains of swine influenza. The origins of this new strain are unknown, and the World Organization for Animal Health (OIE) reports that it has not been isolated in swine. It passes with apparent ease from human to human, an ability attributed to an as-yet unidentified mutation. The strain in most cases causes only mild symptoms, and the infected person makes a full recovery without requiring medical attention and without the use of antiviral medicines.

2. Background.

The H1N1 form of swine flu is one of the descendants of the "Spanish" flu that caused a devastating pandemic in humans in 1918-1919. The "Spanish" flu pandemic infected one third of the world's population (or around 500 million persons at that time) and caused around 50 million deaths. This flu pandemic in humans was associated with H1N1, thus may reflect a mutation spreading either from swine to humans or from humans to swine. Evidence available from that time is not sufficient to resolve this question.

As well as persisting in pigs, the descendants of the 1918 virus have also circulated in humans through the 20th century, contributing to the normal seasonal epidemics of influenza. However, direct transmission from pigs to humans is rare, with 12 cases in the U.S. since 2005.

3. The 1957 "Asian Flu" Pandemic.

The Asian flu was a category 2 flu pandemic outbreak of avian influenza that originated in China in early 1956 and lasted until 1958. It originated from a mutation in flu in wild ducks combining with a pre-existing human strain. The virus was first identified in Guizhou, China. It spread to Singapore in February 1957, reached Hong Kong by April, and the United States by June.

In the United States, this pandemic infected some 45 million Americans and killed approximately 69,800. Estimates of worldwide infection rate varies widely depending on source, ranging from 1 million to 4 million.

Asian Flu was of the H2N2 strain of type A influenza,

and a influenza vaccine was developed in 1957 to contain its outbreak.

The Asian Flu strain later evolved via antigenic shift into H3N2, which caused a milder pandemic from 1968 to 1969.

Both the H2N2 and H3N2 pandemic strains contained avian influenza virus RNA segments. "While the pandemic human influenza viruses of 1957 (H2N2) and 1968 (H3N2) clearly arose through reassortment between human and avian viruses, the influenza virus causing the 'Spanish' flu in 1918 appears to be entirely derived from an avian source." (Belshe, 2005)

4. The 1968-1969 "Hong Kong Flu" Pandemic.

Eleven years after the Asian Flu, the Hong Kong flu pandemic afflicted 50 million Americans.

The Hong Kong Flu was a category 2 flu pandemic caused by a strain of H3N2 descended from H2N2 by antigenic shift, in which genes from multiple subtypes reassorted to form a new virus. This pandemic of 1968 and 1969 killed an estimated one million people worldwide. The pandemic infected an estimated 500,000 Hong Kong residents, 15% of the population, with a low death rate. In the United States, approximately 33,800 people died.

Both the H2N2 and H3N2 pandemic flu strains contained genes from avian influenza viruses. The new subtypes arose in pigs coinfected with avian and human viruses and were soon transferred to humans. Swine were considered the original "intermediate host" for influenza because they supported reassortment of divergent subtypes. However, other hosts — including many bird species — appear capable of similar coinfection, and direct transmission of avian viruses to humans is well known to be possible. H1N1 may have been transmitted directly from birds to humans.

The Hong Kong flu strain shared internal genes and the

neuraminidase with the 1957 Asian Flu. Accumulated anti-bodies to the neuraminidase or internal proteins may have resulted in much fewer casualties than most pandemics. However, cross-immunity within and between subtypes of influenza is poorly understood.

The Hong Kong flu was the first known outbreak of the H3N2 strain, though there is evidence of infections in the late 19th century. The first record of the outbreak in Hong Kong appeared on 13 July 1968. The outbreak reached maximum intensity in 2 weeks, lasting 6 weeks in total. The virus was isolated in Queen Mary Hospital. Flu symptoms lasted 4 to 5 days.

By July 1968, extensive outbreaks were reported in Vietnam and Singapore. By September 1968, it reached India, The Philippines, northern Australia, and Europe. That same month, the virus entered California from returning Vietnam War soldiers. It would reach Japan, Africa, and South America by 1969.

"Three strains of Hong Kong influenza virus isolated from humans were compared with a strain isolated from a calf for their ability to cause disease in calves. One of the human strains. A/Aichi/2/68, was detected for five days in a calf, but all three failed to cause signs of disease. Strain A/cal/Duschanbe/55/71 could be detected for seven days and caused an influenza-like illness in calves."

5. The 1976 Swine Flu Outbreak.

In 1976, about a number of U.S. soldiers became infected with swine flu over a period of a few weeks. It started on February 5, 1976, when an army recruit at Fort Dix said he felt tired and weak. He died the next day, and four of his fellow soldiers were soon hospitalized.

Two weeks after his death, health officials announced that swine flu was the cause of death and that this strain of flu appeared to be closely related to the strain involved in the 1918 flu pandemic. Alarmed public-health officials decided that action must be taken to head off another major pandemic, and they urged President Gerald Ford that every person in the U.S. should be vaccinated for the disease.

However, by the end of the month, investigators found that the virus had "mysteriously disappeared," and there were no more signs of swine flu anywhere on the post. There were isolated cases around the U.S., but those cases were supposedly limited to individuals who caught the virus from pigs.

Nevertheless, President Ford received a swine flu vaccination as soon as it was available and pushed for a nationwide innoculation program. The vaccination program, however, was plagued by delays and public relations problems. But on Oct. 1, 1976, the immunization program began, and by Oct. 11, approximately 40 million people, or about 24% of the U.S. population, had received swine flu immunizations.

When three senior citizens died soon after receiving their swine flu shots, there was a media outcry linking the deaths to the immunizations, despite no positive proof. According to science writer Patrick Di Justo, however, by the time the truth was known — that the deaths were not proven to be related to the vaccine — it was too late. "The government had long feared mass panic about swine flu — now they feared mass panic about the swine flu vaccinations." This became a strong setback to the program.

There were reports of Guillain-Barré syndrome, a paralyzing neuromuscular disorder, affecting some people who had received swine flu immunizations. This syndrome is a rare side-effect of influenza vaccines, with an incidence of about one case per million vaccinations. As a result, Di Justo writes that "the public refused to trust a government-operated health program that killed old people and crippled young people." In total, less than 33 percent of the population had been immunized by the end of 1976. The National Influenza Immunization Program was effectively halted on Dec. 16.

Overall, about 500 cases of Guillain-Barré syndrome (GBS), resulting in death from severe pulmonary complications for 25 people, which, according to Dr. P. Haber, were probably caused by an immunopathological reaction to the 1976 vaccine. Other influenza vaccines have not been linked to GBS, though caution is advised for certain individuals, particularly those with a history of GBS. Still, as observed by a participant in the immunization program, the vaccine killed more Americans than the disease did.

6. The Swine Flu in 1988.

In September 1988, a swine flu virus killed one woman in Wisconsin and infected at least hundreds of others. 32-year-old Barbara Ann Wieners was eight months pregnant when she and her husband, Ed, became ill after visiting the hog barn at the Walworth County Fair. Barbara died eight days later, though doctors were able to induce labor and deliver a healthy daughter before she passed away. Her husband recovered from his symptoms.

Influenza-like illnesses were reportedly widespread among the pigs at the fair they had visited, and 76% of the swine exhibitors there tested positive for the swine flu antibody, but no serious illnesses were detected among this group. Additional studies suggested between one and three health care personnel who had contact with the patient developed mild influenza-like illnesses with antibody evidence of swine flu infection.

7. The 2003-2004 Fujian Flu.

Fujian flu refers to flu caused by either a Fujian human flu strain of the H3N2 subtype of the Influenza A virus or a Fujian bird flu strain of the H5N1 subtype of the Influenza A virus. These strains are named after Fujian, a coastal province of the People's Republic of China that is across the Taiwan strait from Taiwan.

A/Fujian (H3N2) human flu (from A/Fujian/411/2002 (H3N2) — like flu virus strains) caused an unusually severe 2003-2004 flu season. This was due to a reassortment event that caused a minor clade to provide a haemagglutinin gene that later became part of the dominant strain in the 2002-2003 flu season. A/Fujian (H3N2) was made part of the trivalent influenza vaccine for the 2004-2005 flu season, and its descendants are still the most common human H3N2 strain.

8. The 2009 Swine Flu Pandemic: Earliest Cases.

The new strain of swine influenza A (H1N1) involved in the 2009 flu outbreak in humans is a reassortment of several strains of influenza A virus subtype H1N1 that are, separately, endemic in humans, endemic in birds, and endemic in swine. Preliminary genetic characterization found that the hemagglutinin (HA) gene was similar to that of swine flu viruses present in United States pigs since 1999, but the neuraminidase (NA) and matrix protein (M) genes resembled versions present in European swine flu isolates. Viruses with this genetic makeup had not previously been found to be circulating in humans or pigs, but there is no formal national surveillance system to determine what viruses are circulating in pigs in the United States. The origins of this new strain remain unknown.

The United States Department of Agriculture researchers

say that while pig vaccination keeps pigs from getting sick, it does not block infection or shedding of the virus.

Dr. Anne Schuchat, interim Deputy Director for CDC Science and Public Health, said that the American cases were found to be made up of genetic elements from four different flu viruses — North American swine influenza, North American avian influenza, human influenza, and swine influenza virus typically found in Asia and Europe — "an unusually mongrelised mix of genetic sequences." Pigs have been shown to act as a potential "mixing vessel" in which reassortment can occur between flu viruses of several species. This new strain appears to be a result of reassortment of human influenza and swine influenza viruses, presumably due to superinfection in an individual human. Influenza viruses readily undergo reassortment due to antigenic shift because their genome is split between eight pieces of RNA.

The current strain of swine flu can adapt to humans and

FIRST U.S. CASES.

• The earliest known human case, 5 year old Edgar Hernandez, was near a pig farm in La Gloria, Veracruz state, Mexico, that raises almost 1 million pigs a year. Residents of La Gloria have long complained about the clouds of flies that are drawn to the so-called "manure lagoons" created by such mega-farms. Edgar Hernandez was thought to be suffering from ordinary influenza, but laboratory testing revealed he had contracted swine flu. The boy went on to make a full recovery.

"If the people who are supposed to be familiar with this didn't know what it was, how will we ever know how my son got it?" Edgar's mother, Maria del Carman Hernandez said.

• La Gloria, Perote, Veracruz is a small community, surrounded by large pig farms. Reports indicate that during February 2009 over 400 persons in the town had flu like symptoms and 2 infants died of "pneumonia."

Juan Rodriguez died of "pneumonia" February 9th at age 7 months.

Yovanni Apolinar died of "pneumonia" March 12th at age 2 months.

• An unidentified mexican toddler contracted swine flu in Brownsville, Texas, United States and died of swine flu April 29th in Houston, Texas, United States at age 23 months.

spread more efficiently than previously known swine H1N1 strains. Moreover, co-infection of H1N1 swine flu and Oseltamivir resistant H1N1 season flu can lead to acquisition of the H274Y mutation by the swine flu via recombination or reassortment. Swine H1N1 with human H1 and N1 have been reported.

The 1918 flu pandemic strain had undergone polymorphism from swine and human H1N1 in all eight pieces of RNA gene segments. Similar swapping of gene segments in humans co-infected with seasonal human influenza and swine H1N1 can lead to rapid evolution.

The new strain of swine influenza A (H1N1) is currently listed by the United States and World Health Organization as a Phase 5 pandemic virus.

ABOUT THE INFLUENZA VIRUS.

The flu virus is perhaps the trickiest known to medical science; it constantly changes form to elude the protective antibodies that the body has developed in response to previous exposures to influenza or to influenza vaccines. Every two or three years, the virus undergoes minor changes. Then, at intervals of roughly a decade, after the bulk of the world's population has developed some level of resistance to these minor changes, it undergoes a major shift that enables it to tear off on yet another pandemic sweep around the world, infecting hundreds of millions of people who suddenly find their antibody defenses outflanked. Even during the Spanish flu pandemic, the initial wave of the disease was relatively mild, while the second wave was highly lethal.

Medical researchers worldwide, recognizing that the swine flu virus might again mutate into something as deadly as the Spanish flu, were carefully watching the latest 2009 outbreak of swine flu and making contingency plans for a possible global pandemic.

1. Classification of Swine Flu.

SIV strains isolated to date have been classified either as Influenzavirus C or one of the various subtypes of the genus Influenzavirus A, specifically subtypes H1N1, H1N2, H3N1, H3N2, and H2N3.

In swine, three influenza A virus subtypes (H1N1, H3N2, and H1N2) are circulating throughout the world. In the United States, the H1N1 subtype was exclusively prevalent among swine populations before 1998; however, since late August 1998, H3N2 subtypes have been isolated from pigs. As of 2004, H3N2 virus isolates in US swine and turkey stocks were triple reassortants, containing genes from human

(HA, NA, and PB1), swine (NS, NP, and M), and avian (PB2 and PA) lineages.

2. Pigs and the Human Influenza Virus.

Avian influenza virus H3N2 is endemic in pigs in China and has been detected in pigs in Vietnam, increasing fears of the emergence of new variant strains. Health experts say pigs can carry human influenza viruses, which can combine (i.e. exchange homologous genome sub-units by genetic reassortment) with H5N1, passing genes and mutating into a form which can pass easily among humans. H3N2 evolved from H2N2 by antigenic shift. In August 2004, researchers in China found H5N1 in pigs.

Nature magazine reported that Chairul Nidom, a virologist at Airlangga University's tropical disease center in Surabaya, East Java, conducted a survey of swine infections with H5N1 in 2005. He tested the blood of 10 apparently healthy pigs housed near poultry farms in West Java, where avian flu had broken out. Five of the pig samples contained the H5N1 virus. The Indonesian government has since found similar results in the same region. Additional tests of 150 pigs outside the area were negative.

PANDEMIC PREPAREDNESS.

1. Pandemic Influenza Phases: What They Mean

In the 2009 revision of the phase descriptions, World Health Organization (WHO) has retained the use of a six-phased approach for easy incorporation of new recommendations and approaches into existing national preparedness and response plans. The grouping and description of pandemic phases have been revised to make them easier to understand, more precise, and based upon observable phenomena. Phases 1-3 correlate with preparedness, including capacity development and response planning activities, while Phases 4-6 clearly signal the need for response and mitigation efforts. Furthermore, periods after the first pandemic wave are elaborated to facilitate post pandemic recovery activities.

In nature, influenza viruses circulate continuously among animals, especially birds. Even though such viruses might theoretically develop into pandemic viruses, in **Phase 1** no viruses circulating among animals have been reported to cause infections in humans.

In **Phase 2** an animal influenza virus circulating among domesticated or wild animals is known to have caused infec-

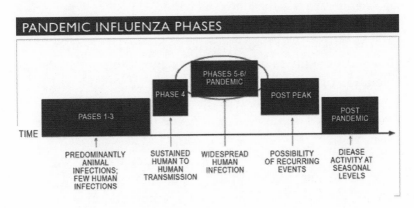

tion in humans, and is therefore considered a potential pandemic threat.

In **Phase 3**, an animal or human-animal influenza reassortant virus has caused sporadic cases or small clusters of disease in people, but has not resulted in human-to-human transmission sufficient to sustain community-level outbreaks. Limited human-to-human transmission may occur under some circumstances, for example, when there is close contact between an infected person and an unprotected caregiver. However, limited transmission under such restricted circumstances does not indicate that the virus has gained the level of transmissibility among humans necessary to cause a pandemic.

Phase 4 is characterized by verified human-to-human transmission of an animal or human-animal influenza reassortant virus able to cause "community-level outbreaks." The ability to cause sustained disease outbreaks in a community marks a significant upwards shift in the risk for a pandemic. Any country that suspects or has verified such an event should urgently consult with WHO so that the situation can be jointly assessed and a decision made by the affected country if implementation of a rapid pandemic containment operation is warranted. Phase 4 indicates a significant increase in risk of a pandemic but does not necessarily mean that a pandemic is a forgone conclusion.

Phase 5 is characterized by human-to-human spread of the virus into at least two countries in one WHO region. While most countries will not be affected at this stage, the declaration of Phase 5 is a strong signal that a pandemic is imminent and that the time to finalize the organization, communication, and implementation of the planned mitigation measures is short.

Phase 6, the pandemic phase, is characterized by community level outbreaks in at least one other country in a different WHO region in addition to the criteria defined in

Phase 5. Designation of this phase will indicate that a global pandemic is under way.

During the **post-peak period**, pandemic disease levels in most countries with adequate surveillance will have dropped below peak observed levels. The post-peak period signifies that pandemic activity appears to be decreasing; however, it is uncertain if additional waves will occur and countries will need to be prepared for a second wave.

Previous pandemics have been characterized by waves of activity spread over months. Once the level of disease activity drops, a critical communications task will be to balance this information with the possibility of another wave. Pandemic waves can be separated by months and an immediate "at-ease" signal may be premature.

In the **post-pandemic period**, influenza disease activity will have returned to levels normally seen for seasonal influenza. It is expected that the pandemic virus will behave as a seasonal influenza A virus. At this stage, it is important to maintain surveillance and update pandemic preparedness and response plans accordingly. An intensive phase of recovery and evaluation may be required.

SWINE FLU: SIGNS, SYMPTOMS, AND DIAGNOSIS.

1. Main Symptoms of Swine Flu in Humans.

According to the Centers for Disease Control and Prevention (CDC), in humans the symptoms of swine flu are similar to those of influenza and of influenza-like illness in general. Symptoms include fever, coughing, sore throat, body aches, headache, chills, and fatigue. The 2009 outbreak has shown an increased percentage of patients reporting diarrhea and vomiting.

Because these symptoms are not specific to swine flu, a differential diagnosis of probable swine flu requires not only symptoms but also a high likelihood of swine flu due to the person's recent history. For example, during the 2009 swine flu outbreak in the United States, CDC advised physicians to "consider swine influenza infection in the differential diagnosis of patients with acute febrile respiratory illness who have either been in contact with persons with confirmed swine flu, or who were in one of the five U.S. states that have reported swine flu cases or in Mexico during the 7 days preceding their illness onset."

Young children may not have typical symptoms, but may have difficulty breathing and low activity. Little is known about how swine flu may affect children. However, the CDC thinks the infection may be similar to other flu infections. Typically, flu infections cause mild disease in children, but children under 5 years old are more likely to have serious illness than older children. Although rare, severe respiratory illness (pneumonia) and deaths have been reported with flu infections in children. Flu infections tend to be more severe in children with chronic medical conditions.

2. Diagnosis.

The swine flu in humans is most contagious during the first five days of the illness although some people, most commonly children, can remain contagious for up to ten days.

A diagnosis of confirmed swine flu requires laboratory testing of a respiratory sample (a simple nose and throat swab) made within the first five days of infection.

PREVENTION.

1. Overview.

Prevention of swine influenza has three components: prevention in swine, prevention of transmission to humans, and prevention of its spread among humans.

2. Prevention in Swine.

Swine influenza has become a greater problem in recent decades as the evolution of the virus has resulted in inconsistent responses to traditional vaccines. Standard commercial swine flu vaccines are effective in controlling the infection when the virus strains match enough to have significant cross-protection, and custom (autogenous) vaccines made from the specific viruses isolated are created and used in the more difficult cases.

Present vaccination strategies for SIV control and prevention in swine farms, typically include the use of one of several bivalent SIV vaccines commercially available in the United States. Of the 97 recent H3N2 isolates examined, only 41 isolates had strong serologic cross-reactions with antiserum to three commercial SIV vaccines. Since the protective ability of influenza vaccines depends primarily on the closeness of the match between the vaccine virus and the epidemic virus, the presence of nonreactive H3N2 SIV variants suggests that current commercial vaccines might not effectively protect pigs from infection with a majority of H3N2 viruses.

3. Prevention of Transmission to Humans.

The easiest way to prevent human transmission is to avoid risk of exposure. The United States has recommended limiting travel to Mexico, where the Swine Flu outbreak started and is in its most advanced state, to essential visits only. However, since the virus has already spread to the United States and other countries, it may be impossible to avoid exposure.

Recommendations to prevent spread of the virus among humans include using standard infection control against influenza. This includes frequent washing of hands with soap and water or with alcohol-based hand sanitizers, especially after being out in public.

Experts agree that hand-washing can help prevent viral infections, including ordinary influenza and the new swine flu virus. Influenza can spread in coughs or sneezes, but an increasing body of evidence shows little particles of virus can linger on tabletops, telephones and other surfaces and be transferred via the fingers to the mouth, nose or eyes. Alcohol-based gel or foam hand sanitizers work well to destroy viruses and bacteria. Anyone with flu-like symptoms such as a sudden fever, cough or muscle aches should stay away from work or public transportation and should see a doctor to be tested.

Social distancing is another tactic. It means staying away from other people who might be infected and can include avoiding large gatherings, spreading out a little at work, or perhaps staying home and lying low if an infection is spreading in a community.

The Centers for Disease Control and Prevention offers these additional tips:

Avoid close contact.
Avoid close contact with people who are sick. When you are sick, keep your distance from others to protect them from getting sick too.

Stay home when you are sick.
If possible, stay home from work, school, and errands

when you are sick. You will help prevent others from catching your illness.

Cover your mouth and nose.
Cover your mouth and nose with a tissue when coughing or sneezing. It may prevent those around you from getting sick.

Clean your hands.
Washing your hands often will help protect you from germs.

Avoid touching your eyes, nose or mouth.
Germs are often spread when a person touches something that is contaminated with germs and then touches his or her eyes, nose, or mouth.

Practice other good health habits.
+

4. A Swine Flu Vaccine.

Although the current influenza vaccine is unlikely to provide protection against the new 2009 H1N1 strain, vaccines against the new strain are being developed and could be ready as early as June 2009.

5. Myths about Spreading Swine Flu.

Swine flu cannot be spread by pork products, since the virus is not transmitted through food. Influenza only spreads between humans through contact with the virus. Coughing and sneezing distributes the virus in the air or on objects or surfaces. It can also be passed by hand when an infected person touches his eyes or mouth, but does not wash them or use a hand sanitizer.

TREATMENT OF SWINE FLU.

1. Antiviral Drugs.

In response to requests from the U.S. Centers for Disease Control and Prevention, on April 27, 2009 the FDA issued Emergency Use Authorizations to make available diagnostic and therapeutic tools to identify and respond to the swine influenza virus under certain circumstances. The agency issued these EUAs for the use of certain Relenza and Tamiflu antiviral drugs, and for the rRT-PCR Swine Flu Panel diagnostic test.

The CDC recommends the use of Tamiflu (oseltamivir) or Relenza (zanamivir) for the treatment and/or prevention of infection with swine influenza viruses, however, the majority of people infected with the virus make a full recovery without requiring medical attention or antiviral drugs. The virus isolates that have been tested from the US and Mexico are however resistant to amantadine and rimantadine. If a person gets sick, antiviral drugs can make the illness milder and make the patient feel better faster. They may also prevent serious flu complications. For treatment, antiviral drugs work best if started soon after getting sick (within 2 days of symptoms).

Some countries have issued orders to stockpile antivirals. These typically have an expiry date of five years after manufacturing.

2. Stockpile Emergency Supplies.

To maintain a secure household during a pandemic flu, the Water Quality & Health Council recommends keeping as supplies food and bottled water, portable power sources and chlorine bleach as an emergency water purifier and surface sanitizer.

SPECIAL INSTRUCTIONS FOR CHILDREN.

There is no sure-fire way to prevent children from coming into contact with the swine flu virus. But common sense and preparedness will go a long way toward helping defend against the swine flu.

1. Tips from the Centers for Disease Control.

- Teach your children to wash their hands frequently with soap and water for 20 seconds. Be sure to set a good example by doing this yourself.
- Teach your children to cough and sneeze into a tissue or into the inside of their elbow. Be sure to set a good example by doing this yourself.
- Teach your children to stay at least six feet away from people who are sick.
- Children who are sick should stay home from school and daycare and stay away from other people until they are better.
- In communities where H1N1 (swine flu) has occurred, stay away from shopping malls, movie theaters, or other places where there are large groups of people.

2. What to do if your child is sick.

- Unless they need medical attention, keep children who are sick at home. Don't send them to school or daycare. Have them drink a lot of liquid (juice, water, Pedialyte ®). Keep the sick child comfortable. Rest is important.
- For fever, sore throat, and muscle aches, you can use

fever-reducing medicines that your doctor recommends based on your child's age. Do not use aspirin with children or teenagers; it can cause Reye's syndrome, a life-threatening illness.

- If someone in your home is sick, keep him or her away from those who are not sick.
- Keep tissues close to the sick person and have a trash bag within reach for disposing used tissues.

If your child comes in contact with someone with H1N1 (swine flu), ask your doctor if he or she should receive antiviral medicines to prevent getting sick from H1N1 (swine flu).

If your child experiences any of the following warning signs, seek emergency medical care:

- Fast breathing or trouble breathing
- Bluish or gray skin color
- Not drinking enough fluids
- Not waking up or not interacting
- Being so irritable that he or she does not want to be held
- Not urinating or no tears when crying
- Their symptoms improve but then return with fever and worse cough

Pathophysiology

Influenza viruses bind through hemagglutinin onto sialic acid sugars on the surfaces of epithelial cells; typically in the nose, throat and lungs of mammals and intestines of birds (Stage 1 in infection figure).

WORLD HEALTH ORGANIZATION REPORT ON SWINE FLU OUTBREAK.

Influenza-like illness in the United States and Mexico

24 April 2009 — The United States Government has reported seven confirmed human cases of Swine Influenza A/H1N1 in the USA (five in California and two in Texas) and nine suspect cases. All seven confirmed cases had mild Influenza-Like Illness (ILI), with only one requiring brief hospitalization. No deaths have been reported.

The Government of Mexico has reported three separate events. In the Federal District of Mexico, surveillance began picking up cases of ILI starting 18 March. The number of cases has risen steadily through April and as of 23 April there are now more than 854 cases of pneumonia from the capital. Of those, 59 have died. In San Luis Potosi, in central Mexico, 24 cases of ILI, with three deaths, have been reported. And from Mexicali, near the border with the United States, four cases of ILI, with no deaths, have been reported.

Of the Mexican cases, 18 have been laboratory confirmed in Canada as Swine Influenza A/H1N1, while 12 of those are genetically identical to the Swine Influenza A/H1N1 viruses from California.

The majority of these cases have occurred in otherwise healthy young adults. Influenza normally affects the very young and the very old, but these age groups have not been heavily affected in Mexico.

Because there are human cases associated with an animal influenza virus, and because of the geographical spread of multiple community outbreaks, plus the somewhat unusual age groups affected, these events are of high concern.

The Swine Influenza A/H1N1 viruses characterized in

this outbreak have not been previously detected in pigs or humans. The viruses so far characterized have been sensitive to oseltamivir, but resistant to both amantadine and rimantadine.

The World Health Organization has been in constant contact with the health authorities in the United States, Mexico and Canada in order to better understand the risk which these ILI events pose. WHO (and PAHO) is sending missions of experts to Mexico to work with health authorities there. It is helping its Member States to increase field epidemiology activities, laboratory diagnosis and clinical management. Moreover, WHO's partners in the Global Alert and Response Network have been alerted and are ready to assist as requested by the Member States.

WHO acknowledges the United States and Mexico for their proactive reporting and their collaboration with WHO and will continue to work with Member States to further characterize the outbreak.

REFERENCES

Heinen PP (15 September 2003). "Swine influenza: a zoonosis." Veterinary Sciences Tomorrow. ISSN 1569-0830. http://www.vetscite.org/publish/articles/000041/print.html. "Influenza B and C viruses are almost exclusively isolated from man, although influenza C virus has also been isolated from pigs and influenza B has recently been isolated from seals."

Maria Zampaglione (April 29, 2009). "Press Release: A/H1N1 influenza like human illness in Mexico and the USA: OIE statement." World Organisation for Animal Health. http://www.oie.int/eng/press/en_090427.htm. Retrieved on April 29, 2009.

http://www.who.int/mediacentre/news/statements/2009/h1n1_20090427/en/index.html

http://www.who.int/csr/disease/swineflu/faq/en/index.html

a b c d Taubenberger JK, Morens DM (2006). "1918 Influenza: the mother of all pandemics." Emerg Infect Dis 12 (1): 15-22. PMID 16494711. http://www.cdc.gov/ncidod/eid/vol12no01/05-0979.htm.

a b c "Soft evidence and hard sell." *New York Times*. 5 September 1976. http://select.nytimes.com/gst/abstract.html?res=F10914FA3E5E14768FDDAC0894D1405B868BF1D3&scp=9&sq=Swine+Flu+epidemic&st=p.

"U.S. pork groups urge hog farmers to reduce flu risk." Reuters. 26 April 2009. http://www.reuters.com/article/latestCrisis/idUSN26488473.

a b "The Last Great Swine Flu Epidemic," Salon.com, April 28, 2009

Heinen PP (15 September 2003). "Swine influenza: a zoonosis." Veterinary Sciences Tomorrow. ISSN 1569-0830. http://www.vetscite.org/publish/articles/000041/print.html. "Influenza B and C viruses are almost exclusively isolated from man, although influenza C virus has also been isolated from pigs and influenza B has recently been isolated from seals."

a b c "Swine Influenza." Swine Diseases (Chest). Iowa State University College of Veterinary Medicine. http://www.vetmed.iastate.edu/departments/vdpam/swine/diseases/chest/swineinfluenza/.

Shin JY, Song MS, Lee EH, Lee YM, Kim SY, Kim HK, Choi JK, Kim CJ, Webby RJ, Choi YK (2006). "Isolation and characterization of novel H3N1 swine influenza viruses from pigs with respiratory diseases in Korea." *Journal of Clinical Microbiology* 44 (11): 3923-7. doi:10.1128/JCM.00904-06. PMID 16928961.

Ma W, Vincent AL, Gramer MR, Brockwell CB, Lager KM, Janke BH, Gauger PC, Patnayak DP, Webby RJ, Richt JA (26 December 2007). "Identification of H2N3 influenza A viruses from swine in the United States." Proc Nat Acad Sci USA 104 (52): 20949-54. doi:10.1073/pnas.0710286104. PMID 18093945. PMC: 2409247. http://www.pnas.org/content/104/52/20949.full.

Yassine HM, Al-Natour MQ, Lee CW, Saif YM (November 2007). "Interspecies and intraspecies transmission of triple reassortant H3N2 influenza A viruses." Virol J 28 (4): 129. doi:10.1186/1743-422X-4-129. PMID 18045494.

Yu, H. (March 2008). "Genetic evolution of swine influenza A (H3N2) viruses in China from 1970 to 2006." Journal of Clinical Microbiology 46 (3): 1067. doi:10.1128/JCM.01257-07. PMID 18199784. http://jcm.asm.org/cgi/con-

tent/full/46/3/1067?maxtoshow=&HITS=10&hits=10&RESULTFORMAT=
&fulltext=phylogen-
etic&searchid=1&FIRSTINDEX=230&resourcetype=HWFIG.

"Bird flu and pandemic influenza: what are the risks?" UK Department of
Health.
http://www.dh.gov.uk/en/Aboutus/MinistersandDepartmentLeaders/ChiefM
edicalOfficer/Features/DH_4102997.

Lindstrom Stephen E, Cox Nancy J, Klimov Alexander (15 October 2004). "Genetic analysis of human H2N2 and early H3N2 influenza viruses, 1957-
1972: evidence for genetic divergence and multiple reassortment events."
Virology 328 (1): 101-19. doi:10.1016/j.virol.2004.06.009. PMID
15380362.

World Health Organization (28 October 2005). "H5N1 avian influenza: timeline"
(PDF). http://www.who.int/csr/disease/avian_influ-
enza/Timeline_28_10a.pdf.

"Indonesian pigs have avian flu virus; bird cases double in China." University of
Minnesota: Center for Infectious Disease Research & Policy. 27 May 2005.
http://www.cidrap.umn.edu/cidrap/content/influ-
enza/avianflu/news/may2705avflu.html. Retrieved on 2009-04-26.

"H5N1 virus may be adapting to pigs in Indonesia." University of Minnesota:
Center for Infectious Disease Research & Policy. 31 March 2009.
http://www.cidrap.umn.edu/cidrap/content/influ-
enza/avianflu/news/mar3109swine-jw.html. Retrieved on 2009-04-26. report on pigs as carriers

Centers for Disease Control and Prevention > Key Facts about Swine Influenza
(Swine Flu) Retrieved on April 27, 2009

"Swine Flu and You." CDC. 2009-04-26.
http://www.cdc.gov/swineflu/swineflu_you.htm. Retrieved on 2009-04-26.

a b Centers for Disease Control and Prevention (April 26, 2009). "CDC Health
Update: Swine Influenza A (H1N1) Update: New Interim Recommendations
and Guidance for Health Directors about Strategic National Stockpile Ma-
teriel." Health Alert Network.
http://www.cdc.gov/swineflu/HAN/042609.htm. Retrieved on April 27,
2009.

"Swine flu virus turns endemic." National Hog Farmer. 15 September 2007.
http://nationalhogfarmer.com/mag/swine_flu_virus_endemic/.

"Swine." Custom Vaccines. Novartis. http://www.live-
stock.novartis.com/cv_swine.html.

Gramer Marie René, Lee Jee Hoon, Choi Young Ki, Goyal Sagar M, Joo Han
Soo (July 2007). "Serologic and genetic characterization of North American
H3N2 swine influenza A viruses." Canadian Journal of Veterinary Research
71 (3): 201-206. PMID 1899866.
http://www.pubmedcentral.nih.gov/articlerender.fcgi?artid=1899866.

Myers KP, Olsen CW, Gray GC (April 2007). "Cases of swine influenza in humans: a review of the literature." Clin Infect Dis 44 (8): 1084-8.
doi:10.1086/512813. PMID 17366454.

"Q & A: Key facts about swine influenza (swine flu) — Spread of Swine Flu."
Centers for Disease Control and Prevention. 24 April 2009.
http://www.cdc.gov/swineflu/key_facts.htm. Retrieved on 2009-04-26.

"Q & A: Key facts about swine influenza (swine flu) — Diagnosis." Centers for Disease Control and Prevention. 24 April 2009. http://www.cdc.gov/swineflu/key_facts.htm. Retrieved on 2009-04-26.

"CDC—Influenza (Flu) | Swine Influenza (Flu) Investigation." Cdc.gov. http://cdc.gov/swineflu/investigation.htm. Retrieved on 2009-04-27.

"Q & A: Key facts about swine influenza (swine flu) — Virus Strains." Centers for Disease Control and Prevention. 24 April 2009. http://www.cdc.gov/swineflu/key_facts.htm. Retrieved on 2009-04-26.

Lauren Petty (April 28, 2009). "Swine Flu Vaccine Could Be Ready in 6 Weeks." NBC Connecticut. http://www.nbcconnecticut.com/news/local/CT-Company-Making-Swine-Flu-Vaccine.html. Retrieved on April 28, 2009.

FDA Authorizes Emergency Use of Influenza Medicines, Diagnostic Test in Response to Swine Flu Outbreak in Humans. FDA News, April 27, 2009.

http://www.who.int/csr/disease/swineflu/faq/en/index.html

"Antiviral Drugs and Swine Influenza." Centers for Disease Control. http://www.cdc.gov/swineflu/antiviral_swine.htm. Retrieved on 2009-04-27.

www.waterandhealth.org/flu/drralph_checklist.pdf "What will you need to stay healthy and secure during a pendemic flu outbreak?" WaterandHealth.org. www.waterandhealth.org/flu/drralph_checklist.pdf. Retrieved on 2009-04-28.

"DA probes reported swine flu 'outbreak' in N. Ecija." Gmanews.tv. http://www.gmanews.tv/story/56805/DA-probes-reported-swine-flu-outbreak-in-N-Ecija. Retrieved on 2009-04-25.

"Gov't declares hog cholera alert in Luzon." Gmanews.tv. http://www.gmanews.tv/story/53014/Govt-declares-hog-cholera-alert-in-Luzon. Retrieved on 2009-04-25.

Wagner, R; Matrosovich M, Klenk H (May-June 2002). "Functional balance between haemagglutinin and neuraminidase in influenza virus infections." Reviews in Medical Virology 12 (3): 159-66. doi:10.1002/rmv.352. PMID 11987141.

International Committee on Taxonomy of Viruses. "The Universal Virus Database, version 4: Influenza A." http://www.ncbi.nlm.nih.gov/ICTVdb/ICTVdB/00.046.0.01.htm.

a b Gray GC, Kayali G (April 2009). "Facing pandemic influenza threats: the importance of including poultry and swine workers in preparedness plans." Poultry Science 88 (4): 880-4. doi:10.3382/ps.2008-00335. PMID 19276439.

Gray GC, McCarthy T, Capuano AW, Setterquist SF, Olsen CW, Alavanja MC (December 2007). "Swine workers and swine influenza virus infections." Emerging Infectious Diseases 13 (12): 1871-8. PMID 182580381 http://www.cdc.gov/eid/content/13/12/1871.htm.

"Deadly new flu virus in US and Mexico may go pandemic." New Scientist. 2009-04-24. http://www.newscientist.com/article/dn17025-deadly-new-flu-virus-in-us-and-mexico-may-go-pandemic.html. Retrieved on 2009-04-26.

"Q & A: Key facts about swine influenza (swine flu)—Symptoms." Centers for Disease Control and Prevention. 24 April 2009. http://www.cdc.gov/swineflu/key_facts.htm. Retrieved on 2009-04-26.

Schmeck, Harold M. (March 25, 1976). "Ford Urges Flu Campaign To Inoculate Entire U.S." New York Times. http://select.nytimes.com/gst/abstract.html?res=F50A17FD3C5A167493C7AB1788D85F428785F9.

Richard E. Neustadt and Harvey V. Fineberg. (1978). The Swine Flu Affair: Decision-Making on a Slippery Disease. National Academies Press.

Vellozzi C, Burwen DR, Dobardzic A, Ball R, Walton K, Haber P (March 2009). "Safety of trivalent inactivated influenza vaccines in adults: Background for pandemic influenza vaccine safety monitoring." *Vaccine* 27 (15): 2114-2120. doi:10.1016/j.vaccine.2009.01.125. PMID 19356614.

Haber P, Sejvar J, Mikaeloff Y, Destefano F (2009). "Vaccines and Guillain-Barré syndrome." Drug Saf 32 (4): 309-23. doi:10.2165/00002018-200932040-00005 (inactive 2009-04-26). PMID 19388722.

"Influenza / Flu Vaccine." University of Illinois at Springfield. http://www.uis.edu/healthservices/immunizations/influenzavaccine.html. Retrieved on 26 April 2009.

BBC: The World; April 28, 2009.

http://www.cdc.gov/swineflu/key_facts.htm Key Facts About Swine Flu (CDC)

Jason George (April 28, 2009). "Swine flu: Last U.S. swine flu death in 1988 in Wisconsin." Chicago Tribune. http://www.chicagotribune.com/news/local/chi-wisconsin-swine-fluapr28,0,1940041.story.

"Swine influenza A (H1N1) infection in two children — Southern California, March—April 2009." Morbidity and Mortality Weekly Report. Centers for Disease Control. 22 April 2009. http://www.cdc.gov/mmwr/preview/mmwrhtml/mm5815a5.htm.

http://blogs.wsj.com/health/2009/04/29/search-for-swine-flus-patient-zero-leads-to-mexican-boy/

Mexico outbreak traced to 'manure lagoons' at pig farm, Times Online, April 28, 2009

"Swine flu: The predictable pandemic?" 2009-04-29. http://www.newscientist.com/article/mg20227063.800-swine-flu-the-predictable-pandemic.html?full=true/.

"Deadly new flu virus in US and Mexico may go pandemic." *New Scientist.* 2009-04-26. http://www.newscientist.com/article/dn17025-deadly-new-flu-virus-in-us-and-mexico-may-go-pandemic.html. Retrieved on 2009-04-26.

Robert Roos (2007-12-20). "New swine flu virus supports 'mixing vessel' theory." http://www.cidrap.umn.edu/cidrap/content/influenza/avianflu/news/dec2007swine.html.

"Identification of H2N3 influenza A viruses from swine in the United States." 2007-12-26. doi:10.1073/pnas.0710286104. http://www.pnas.org/content/104/52/20949.abstract.

"Human Transmission of Swine H1N1 in Southern California." 2007-04-22. http://www.recombinomics.com/News/04220902/H1N1_CA_Swine_H2H.html.

"Human Transmission of Swine H1N1 in Southern California." 2007-04-22. http://www.recombinomics.com/News/04220902/H1N1_CA_Swine_H2H.html.

"Human Transmission of Swine H1N1 in Southern California." 2007-04-22. http://www.recombinomics.com/News/04220902/H1N1_CA_Swine_H2H.html.

"WHO raises H1N1 Virus to Phase 5—Pandemic Emminent." 2009-04-29. http://politicolnews.com/who-raises-h1n1-to-stage-5/. a b c Starling, Arthur

(2006). Plague, SARS, and the Story of Medicine in Hong Kong. HK University Press. p. 55. ISBN 9622098053. http://books.google.com/books?id=WBx6McA35iYC.

U.S. Department of Health and Human Services, http://www.pandemicflu.gov/general/historicaloverview.html

Chapter Two : Avian Influenza by Timm C. Harder and Ortrud Werner from the on-line Book *Influenza Report 2006*.

J Infect Dis. 1977 Apr;135(4):678-80. article "Strains of Hong Kong Influenza Virus in Calves."

"Avian influenza frequently asked questions." World Health Organization. December 5, 2005. http://www.who.int/csr/disease/avian_influenza/avian_faqs/en/. Retrieved on 2009-02-13. "A pandemic can start when three conditions have been met: a new influenza virus subtype emerges; it infects humans, causing serious illness; and it spreads easily and sustainably among humans".

"Ancient Athenian Plague Proves to Be Typhoid." Scientific American. January 25, 2006.

Past pandemics that ravaged Europe. BBC News, November 7. 2005

Cambridge Catalogue page "Plague and the End of Antiquity."

Quotes from book "Plague and the End of Antiquity" Lester K. Little, ed., Plague and the End of Antiquity: The Pandemic of 541-750, Cambridge, 2006. ISBN 0-521-84639-0

The History of the Bubonic Plague

Death on a Grand Scale

Plague—Love To Know 1911

"A List of National Epidemics of Plague in England 1348-1665"

Jo Revill. "Black Death blamed on man, not rats | UK news | *The Observer.*" The Observer. http://www.guardian.co.uk/uk/2004/may/16/health.books. Retrieved on 2008-11-03.

Plague. World Health Organization.

Cholera- Biological Weapons

The 1832 Cholera Epidemic in New York State

Asiatic Cholera Pandemic of 1826-37

The Cholera Epidemic Years in the United States

Cholera's seven pandemics, cbc.ca, December 2, 2008

a b The 1832 Cholera Epidemic in New York State—Page 2. By G. William Beardslee

Asiatic Cholera Pandemic of 1846-63 . UCLA School of Public Health.

Eastern European Plagues and Epidemics 1300-1918

Cholera—Love To Know 1911

"The cholera in Spain." *New York Times*. 1890-06-20. http://query.nytimes.com/gst/abstract.html?res=9E05EED7123BE533A25753C2A9609C94619ED7CF. Retrieved on 2008-12-08.

Barry, John M. (2004). The Great Influenza: The Epic Story of the Greatest Plague in History. Viking Penguin. ISBN 0-670-89473-7.

cholera :: Seven pandemics, Britannica Online Encyclopedia

1900s: The Epidemic Years, Society of Philippine Health History

50 Years of Influenza Surveillance. World Health Organization.

"Pandemic Flu." Department of Health and Social Security.

Beveridge, W.I.B. (1977) Influenza: The Last Great Plague: An Unfinished Story of Discovery, New York: Prodist. ISBN 0-88202-118-4.

Potter, C.W. (October 2001). "A History of Influenza." Journal of Applied Microbiology 91 (4): 572-579. doi:10.1046/j.1365-2672.2001.01492.x. http://www.blackwell-synergy.com/doi/abs/10.1046/j.1365-2672.2001.01492.x. Retrieved on 2006-08-20.

"Bird flu timeline: A history of influenza from 412 BC - AD 2006." NaturalNews.

CIDRAP article Pandemic Influenza Last updated 29 May 2008

Taubenberger JK, Morens DM (January 2006). "1918 Influenza: the mother of all pandemics." Emerg Infect Dis (Centers for Disease Control and Prevention (CDC)) 12 (1). http://www.cdc.gov/ncidod/eid/vol12no01/05-0979.htm.

Spanish flu, ScienceDaily

Pandemics and Pandemic Threats since 1900. U.S. Department of Health & Human Services

Q&A: Swine flu. BBC News. April 27, 2009.

"World health group issues alert Mexican president tries to isolate those with swine flu." Associate Press. April 25, 2009. http://www.jsonline.com/news/usandworld/43705182.html. Retrieved on 2009-04-26.

War and Pestilence, TIME

See a large copy of the chart here: http://www.adept-plm.com/Newsletter/NapoleonsMarch.htm, but discussed at length in Edward Tufte, The Visual Display of Quantitative Information (London: Graphics Press, 1992)

a b Joseph M. Conlon. "The historical impact of epidemic typhus" (PDF). http://entomology.montana.edu/historybug/TYPHUS-Conlon.pdf.

Soviet Prisoners of War: Forgotten Nazi Victims of World War II By Jonathan Nor, TheHistoryNet

The virus reached the U.S. by way of Haiti, genetic study shows. Los Angeles Times. October 30, 2007.

The South African Department of Health Study, 2006

AIDS Toll May Reach 100 Million in Africa. Washington Post. June 4, 2006.

Aids could kill 90 million Africans, says UN

Smallpox and Vaccinia. National Center for Biotechnology Information.

"UC Davis Magazine, Summer 2006: Epidemics on the Horizon." http://ucdavismagazine.ucdavis.edu/issues/su06/feature_1b.html. Retrieved on 2008-01-03.

How Poxviruses Such As Smallpox Evade The Immune System, ScienceDaily, February 1, 2008

"Smallpox." WHO Factsheet. Retrieved on 2007-09-22.

De Cock KM (2001). "(Book Review) The Eradication of Smallpox: Edward Jenner and The First and Only Eradication of a Human Infectious Disease." Nature Medicine 7: 15-6. doi:10.1038/83283. http://www.nature.com/nm/journal/v7/n1/full/nm0101_15b.html.

Center for Disease Control & National Immunization Program. Measles History, article online 2001. Available from http://www.cdc.gov.nip/diseases/measles/history.htm

a b Torrey EF and Yolken RH. 2005. Their bugs are worse than their bite. Wash-

ington Post, April 3, p. B01.

"The global burden of measles in the year 2000—a model that uses country-specific indicators." Global Programme on Evidence for Health Policy, World Health Organization.

Man and Microbes: Disease and Plagues in History and Modern Times; by Arno Karlen

"Measles and Small Pox as an Allied Army of the Conquistadors of America" by Carlos Ruvalcaba, translated by Theresa M. Betz in "Encounters" (Double Issue No. 5-6, pp. 44-45)

Smallpox: Eradicating the Scourge

Smallpox The Fight to Eradicate a Global Scourge, David A. Koplow

"The first smallpox epidemic on the Canadian Plains: In the fur-traders' words", National Institutes of Health

The Story Of . . . Smallpox — and other Deadly Eurasian Germs

Stacy Goodling, "Effects of European Diseases on the Inhabitants of the New World"

Smallpox Through History

New Zealand Historical Perspective

How did Easter Island's ancient statues lead to the destruction of an entire ecosystem?, The Independent

Fiji School of Medicine

Measles hits rare Andaman tribe. BBC News. May 16, 2006.

Meeting the First Inhabitants, TIMEasia.com, 8/21/2000

Genetic Study Bolsters Columbus Link to Syphilis, *New York Times*, January 15, 2008

Columbus May Have Brought Syphilis to Europe, LiveScience

"Sahib: The British Soldier in India, 1750-1914 by Richard Holmes"

Dr. Francisco de Balmis and his Mission of Mercy, Society of Philippine Heath History

Lewis Cass and the Politics of Disease: The Indian Vaccination Act of 1832

Conquest and Disease or Colonialism and Health?, Gresham College | Lectures and Events

WHO Media centre (2001). Fact sheet N°259: African trypanosomiasis or sleeping sickness. http://www.who.int/mediacentre/factsheets/fs259/en/index.html.

The Origins of African Population Growth, by John Iliffe, The Journal of African HistoryVol. 30, No. 1 (1989), pp. 165-169

World Population Clock—Worldometers

World Health Organization (WHO). Tuberculosis Fact sheet N°104—Global and regional incidence. March 2006, Retrieved on 6 October 2006.

Centers for Disease Control. Fact Sheet: Tuberculosis in the United States. 17 March 2005, Retrieved on 6 October 2006.

Multidrug-Resistant Tuberculosis. Centers for Disease Control and Prevention.

Leprosy 'could pose new threat.' BBC News. April 3, 2007.

Leprosy (Hansen's Disease).Centers for Disease Control and Prevention (CDC).

"Leprosy." WHO. http://www.who.int/mediacentre/factsheets/fs101/en/. Retrieved on 2007-08-22.

"Medieval leprosy reconsidered." International Social Science Review, Spring-Summer, 2006, by Timothy S. Miller, Rachel Smith-Savage.

"Leprosy and mortality in the Medieval Danish village of Tirup"

"Leprosy." *Catholic Encyclopedia*. New York: Robert Appleton Company. 1913. http://en.wikisource.org/wiki/Catholic_Encyclopedia_(1913)/Leprosy.

Malaria Facts. Centers for Disease Control and Prevention.

White NJ (April 2004). "Antimalarial drug resistance." J. Clin. Invest. 113 (8): 1084-92. doi:10.1172/JCI21682. PMID 15085184.

Vector- and Rodent-Borne Diseases in Europe and North America. Norman G. Gratz. World Health Organization, Geneva.

"A Brief History of Malaria"

Yellow Fever—Love To Know 1911.

Arnebeck, Bob (January 30, 2008). "A Short History of Yellow Fever in the US." Benjamin Rush, Yellow Fever and the Birth of Modern Medicine. http://www.geocities.com/bobarnebeck/history.html. Retrieved on 04-12-2008.

Tiger mosquitoes and the history of yellow fever and dengue in Spain.

Africa's Nations Start to Be Their Brothers' Keepers. *New York Times*, October 15, 1995.

Health ministers to accelerate efforts against drug-resistant TB. World Health Organization.

Tuberculosis: A new pandemic?. CNN.com

Drug-resistant plague a 'major threat,' say scientists, SciDev.Net

Researchers sound the alarm: the multidrug resistance of the plague bacillus could spread. Pasteur.fr

Klenk et al (2008). "Avian Influenza: Molecular Mechanisms of Pathogenesis and Host Range." Animal Viruses: Molecular Biology. Caister Academic Press. ISBN 978-1-904455-22-6.

Kawaoka Y (editor). (2006). Influenza Virology: Current Topics. Caister Academic Press. ISBN 978-1-904455-06-6. http://www.horizonpress.com/flu.

Wheelis M. (2002), "Biological warfare at the 1346 siege of Caffa." Emerg Infect Dis (Center for Disease Control), http://www.cdc.gov/ncidod/EID/vol8no9/01-0536.htm

Diamond, Jared (1997), Guns, Germs, and Steel: The Fates of Human Societies, W.W. Norton & Company, ISBN 0-393-03891-2

Dixon, Never Come to Peace, 152-55; McConnell, A Country Between, 195-96; Dowd, War under Heaven, 190. For historians who believe the attempt at infection was successful, see Nester, Haughty Conquerors," 112; Jennings, Empire of Fortune, 447-48.

Christopher Hudson (2 March 2007). "Doctors of Depravity" Daily Mail. http://www.dailymail.co.uk/pages/live/articles/news/news.html?in_article_id=439776&in_page_id=1770.

Ken Alibek and S. Handelman. Biohazard: The Chilling True Story of the Largest Covert Biological Weapons Program in the World—Told from Inside by the Man Who Ran it. 1999. Delta (2000) ISBN 0-385-33496-6 [5].

William J Broad, Soviet Defector Says China Had Accident at a Germ Plant, *New York Times*, April 5, 1999

The editor wishes to acknowledge the kind assistance of the World Health Organization, the Centers for Disease Control and Prevention, the National Institute of Health, and other U.S. government agencies through their online resources, as well as the Wikipedia.